Makko Ho

Six simple exercises to bring health and vitality to the whole body

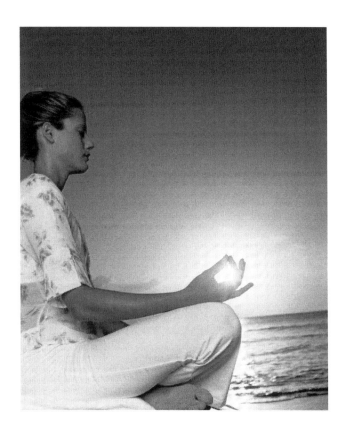

Francine Milford

Makko Ho: Six simple exercises to bring health and vitality to the whole body by Francine Milford

Copyright©2005 Francine Milford and its licensors. All rights reserved.

2013 Updated Edition

All rights reserved. No part of this publication may be reproduced or transmitted in any form or by any means electronic or mechanical, including photocopy, recording, or any information storage and retrieval system, without permission in writing from the copyright owner.

ISBN: 978-1-4116-4335-2

Photographs by Paul, Larry and Francine Milford

Models: Josette Aramini and Francine Milford

Caution

The techniques, ideas, and suggestions presented in this book are not intended as a substitute for proper medical advice. Any application of the techniques, ideas, and suggestions in this book is at the reader's sole discretion and risk.

Sounds Good to Me Publishing

Table of Contents

Chapter One..**page 5**

    What are the Meridians...page 5
    Yin and Yang..page 7
    Five elements and the meridians.......................................page 8
    Element of fire..page 10
    Element of wood...page 11
    Element of water...page 12
    Element of metal...page 13
    Element of wood...page 14

Chapter Two...**page 15**
    The Breath..page 15
    The Breath Technique..page 17

Chapter Three..**page 19**
    The Practice of Makko Ho..page 19

Chapter Four..**page 21**
    Large Intestine and Lung Meridians..................................page 21
    Large Intestine Meridian..page 21
    Lung Meridian..page 24

Chapter Five...**page 31**
    Small Intestine and Heart Meridians.................................page 31
    Small Intestine Meridian..page 31
    Heart Meridian...page 34

Chapter Six..**page 39**
    Bladder and Kidney Meridians...page 39
    Bladder Meridian...page 39
    Kidney Meridian...page 42

Chapter Seven...**page 47**
    Triple Heater and Heart Protector Meridians....................page 47
    Triple Heater Meridian...page 47
    Heart Protector Meridian...page 49

Chapter Eight...**page 51**
    Liver and Gall Bladder Meridians......................................page 51
    Liver Meridian..page 51
    Gall Bladder Meridian..page 54

Chapter Nine..**page 59**
    Spleen and Stomach Meridians...page 59
    Spleen Meridian...page 59
    Stomach Meridian..page 62

Chapter Ten...**page 69**
Finishing Exercise..page 69
The Makko Ho Routine...page 71
Chapter Eleven..**page 75**
The Food Pyramid..page 75
About the Author..**page 81**
References...**page 82**
My Daily Journal..**page 83**

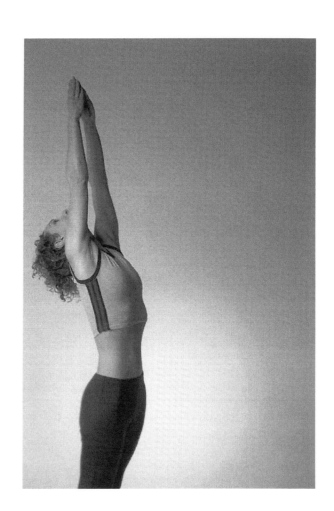

Chapter One
Makko Ho

With their knowledge of the energy pathways of the human body, practitioners in Japan created a set of six simple exercises that would affect every major organ and system in the human body. They called this system, Makko Ho.

Used for centuries in Japan to improve the flow of energy (Qi) in the body, Makko Ho came to the United States in the 1960s. The exercises were widely used in the shiatsu world as a self-healing technique for both the practitioner and the client.

Each of the original six Makko Ho exercises work on a specific "pair" of meridians. Since there are 12 major meridians, or energy pathways, in the human body, that means that there are 6 exercises for these meridians.

Each of these exercises are said to enhance the flow of energy through that meridian as well as to enhance its function. The six exercises include the whole body and all the vital organs.

While performing each of these exercises, it is important to note that just imitating the movements will not be as effective as if you would concentrate and breathe through each movement. You must "feel" into each exercise and bring your awareness to your body and become aware of how your body is responding to each movement.

By becoming more aware of your body and mind's response to movement, you can more effectively alter the perception of each movement. The true benefits of these and other exercises dealing with energy work will be discovered when you have explored then with the right level of focus and attitude.

The Meridians

What are the Meridians?

Meridians are pathways, or channels, of energy that run through the human body. It is said that there are 12 major meridian channels in the body. Each meridian gives direction to the flow of energy. The energy flow is perceived as yin or yang.

Each of the twelve main meridians corresponds to an organ of the body.
Even though each meridian is named for an organ in the body, it is not the organ that is of particular interest, but the PROCESS of the energy flow through that organ and through the rest of the body. In this way, instead of concentrating on the flow of energy in one organ, we are concerned with the flow of energy throughout the entire person and the balance of that energy.

When the flow of energy passes through the human body free and unhampered by blockages, there is a balance, a homeostasis that is formed. It is imbalances and blockages that may lead to physical, mental, and even spiritual problems in the body. If left untreated, these problems could become very serious and lead to the failure of the other systems in the body.

This is why it is important to "catch" the small problems early on, before they become large problems and affect the rest of the body.

Keeping your meridians unblocked and balanced will help to support your immune system. This in turn will help to enhance your ability to fight disease. In this state of balance, you will also be able to pick up the subtle early warning signs of an impending illness and be able to counteract its effects with preventative health care. Impending illnesses such as colds, flu, stress, headaches, etc. are all signs of a body that is being overstressed. Catching these and other symptoms in the early stages can save you from being the victim of a full blown attack.

Sometimes, recognizing the early symptoms can help you to stop the impeding illness in its tracks, before it even has a change to take hold in your body.

Now isn't that something worth exercising for?

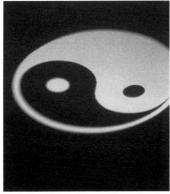

The Yin Yang Symbol

Yin and Yang

In the world of duality, there is Yin and Yang. 'Yin' represents the feminine, the receiver. 'Yang' represents the masculine, the sender. In addition to each of the meridians of the body being dominated by either Yin or Yang (female or masculine energy), each meridian is also associated with one of the five elements. The five elements are earth, fire, water, metal and wood. In some books you will see some differences in the five elements. For this book we will concentrate on the five elements that I have listed.

The path that the energy flow takes through each of the meridians is either in an ascending or descending direction. Yin meridians flow upwards and Yang meridians flow downwards.

The Upper Yin Meridians - Travels from the chest to the tips of the fingers.

Heart

Lung

Circulation-Sex

The Upper Yang Meridians - Travels from the tips of the fingers to the head

Small Intestine

Triple Warmer

Large Intestine

The Lower Yin Meridians - Travels from the tips of the toes to the chest

Spleen

Live

Kidney

The Lower Yang Meridians - Travels from the head to the tips of the toes

Stomach Gall

Bladder

Bladder

The Five Elements and the Meridians

Each pair of meridians are also related to a specific "Element". These elements will be discussed later on in the book as they are associated with a paired meridian system.

With regards to the Makko ho exercises, it is important for the practitioner to think of the property of the element that they are working with. For instance,

When working with fire, you would think of flames, heat and warmth. You would also think of the sun, of a fire, or maybe even an oven. These images should spark vitality, life, power and the colors red and orange-red.

When working with water you may think of the color of blue and think of coolness, or refreshment. You may have feelings of fluidity and easy movement like a babbling brook or moving river. When imagining the elements, it is your perception that counts.

The Five Elements:

Fire

Wood

Water

Metal

Earth

The Five elements and their paired meridians are as follows:

Bladder and Kidneys Water

*

Triple Heart Warmer and Protector Fire

*

Lungs and Large Intestine Metal & Air

*

Heart and Small Intestine Fire

*

Liver and Gall Bladder Wood

*

Spleen and Stomach Earth

*

The Element of Fire

Fire represents the heart.

Fire corresponds with OPENING - (such as in unconditional giving, experiencing joy, showing compassion, and sharing with others).

Too much fire can lead to self-detriment with little or no sense of limits and boundaries in relationships. Too much fire may lead to an inability to give emotionally. A fire personal can be Non spontaneous.

Fire is supported by trusting and is controlled by aligning

A Fire person is one who is emotional, communicative, and articulate. They tend to be very sociable, loving, and can be quite spiritual in outlook.

Additional attributes of the Fire Element include:

- Relief and Joy and Hysteria
- Season is Summer
- Yang
- Adolescence (turbulence)
- Growth
- 11 a.m.-3 p.m.
- 7 p.m.-11 p.m.
- Flavor is Bitterness
- Direction is South
- Associated with the Tongue
- Sense is Speech
- Sound of the Voice is Laughter
- Associated with the Blood Vessels
- Scent is Burnt or Scorched
- Dreams of laughter, fear or fire
- Number is 7
- Musical Note is Sol
- Color is Red
- Mind Spirit Watching

The Element of Wood

Wood is expressed in the idea of trusting. Specifically means trusting God, the Universe Flow, and the Great Spirit. It focuses on intent, doing your best and transcending limitations, both inwardly and outwardly.

Too much wood can lead to timidness, depression, being overly cautious, lack of focus, running on empty, impulsiveness, etc. Wood is long lasting anger.

It is the rising, expanding, and growing feeling we are aware of in the spring when nature awakens from the long sleep of winter and the great surge of activity and growth that starts the year begins. A wood person is creative, hardworking, decisive, and directing. Wood likes to be in control and to keep busy.

Additional attributes of the Wood Element include:

- 11p.m.-3 a.m.
- Direction is east
- Season is spring
- Flavor is Sour
- Associated with the Eyes
- Sense is Sight
- Sound of Voice is shouting
- Part of the Body is the Tendons and Muscles
- Scent is Sour-Sour Sweet
- Taste is Sour
- Germination
- Dreams of trees or hostilities
- Number is 8
- Musical note is Me
- Color is Green
- Soul
- Anger
- Assertiveness
- Walking

The Element of Water

Water likes to set foundations, maintain integrity and balance and to gather and store energy for reserves. Water is the ability to keep rooted in the midst of chaos, a rudder in the flow of life. Water is the optimal response to life - no judgments, no preconceptions, no panic.

Too much water can lead to a lack of direction, not completing things, extremism, fear, or fixation on one way of doing things.

Water people are flexible, well-motivated, and ambitious. They can all tend to be lazy and "go with the flow" too much.

Additional attributes of the Water Element include:

- 3 p.m.-7 p.m.
- Direction is north
- Season is winter
- Flavor is Salty
- Associated with the Ears
- Sense if Hearing
- Sounds of the Voice is Groaning or Moaning
- Part of the Body is the Bones and Teeth
- Scent is Putrid, fish
- Storing
- Dreams of water and boast and swimming
- Number is 6
- Musical Note is La
- Color is Black (or Blue)
- Will
- Fear
- Courage
- Standing
- Head Hair

Element of Metal

Metal (gold), deals with the lungs and reflects releasing. Metal steps back from an experience and evaluates and sorts it out. Metal refines goals and directions and the ability to let go of excessive emotional attachments to people and events. Metal is inspiration, acknowledging self and others and refining one's character.

Too much metal leads to chronic grieving and sadness. It also can lead to aloofness, obsessiveness, living in the past or extreme attachments.

A Metal person is well-organized, neat, methodical, and meticulous. They tend to be very self-contained and do not express emotion much. Metal is the consolidation of our achievements, a sense of positivity about a situation.

Additional attributes of the Metal Element include:

• 3 a.m.-7 a.m.
• Direction is west
• Season is autumn
• Flavor is Spicy
• Associated with the nose
• Sense is Smell
• Sound of the Voice is weeping
• Part of the body is the skin and hair
• Scent is Pungent or Spicy
• Reaping
• Dreams of white or metallic objects, murder, flying
• Number is 9
• Color is White
• Body or Animal spirit
• Sadness
• Empathy
• Lying Down
• Skin and body hair

Element of Earth

Earth corresponds to the Spleen and is associated with Connecting. Earth is patience, being in the moment, focusing thought and attention, making useful mental associations. Earth represents stability, home, service, and a taste for life.

Too much earth can lead to obsessiveness, inability to be in the moment, and acting scattered brained. It can also lead to acting distracted (not present), lack of awareness of surroundings, and difficulty in moving. Self-pity, yang turned yin, and maturity of our reproductive years.

An Earth person is sympathetic, considerate, and supportive. They tend to be an "earth mother" type, with focus on caring for others.

Additional attributes of the Earth Element include:

- 7 a.m.-11 a.m.
- Direction is Venter
- Flavor is Sweet
- Associated with the Mouth
- Sense is Touch
- Sound of Voice is Singing
- Part of the body is the large muscles and limbs
- Scent is Sweet
- Transformation
- Dreams of being overweight or of starvation. Dreams of construction, music, hills or marshes
- Number is 5
- Color is Yellow
- Thought
- Worry
- Concern
- Sitting
- Lips

Chapter Two
  The Breath

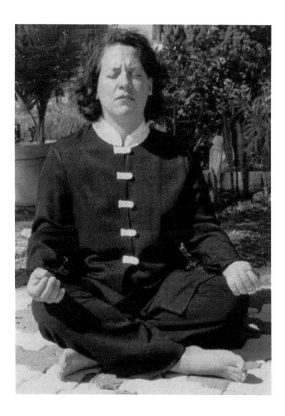

Breathing is vital to any eastern exercise routine. By following correct breathing techniques and working within your body's physical limitations, you will see results within two weeks.

Some results may be as simple as just feeling more relaxed and at peace with the world. Other changes you may experience can be improvement in limited mobility, increased circulation, better sleeping, and yes, even weight loss.

Since everyone is coming to the exercise program with a different set of values and physical and mental programming, it is important not to chart your progress by someone else's standards. We are all unique beings and results that one person may be having will be quite different from results that someone else will be experiences. Be patient.

With consistent encouragement and daily practice, you will achieve all that you are capable of achieving. Don't give up! And now, we will talk about the breath.

From now on, make a promise to yourself. For at least 5 minutes a day, sit with yourself and breathe. You can find this five minutes in any part of your day, even while watching your favorite program on television. Just press the 'mute' button on your channel changer and breathe through the commercials.

There are many, many different forms of breathing. If you are interested in pursuing more techniques for using your breath, then you may want to purchase one of my upcoming books on breath work. But until then, we will practice this one simple and easy to use breathing technique that is guaranteed to make you feel more relaxed and calmer in just minutes.

If you should feel dizzy after performing this technique, don't panic. It is quite natural for westerners who have been chest breathing all of their lives to become dizzy from deep breathing. With practice, this too will pass.

I became quite discouraged when I began deep breathing. It always made me dizzy, and then I would quit. I would try again, become frustrated, and quit. It took me two years before I got the hang of it and it was worth every day I struggled. I promise.

Now, turn off the telephone, computer and television. The next five minutes is just for you and your body. Find a comfortable place to sit or lie down and allow yourself five minutes of uninterrupted peace.

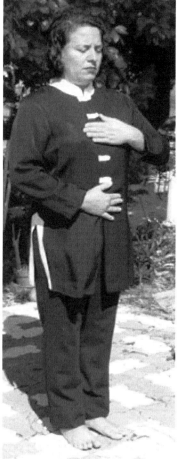

The Breath Technique

The Breath Technique

1. Place your left hand in the middle of your chest, just above your breast. Place your right hand on your stomach, just below the ribcage.

2. Now take a breath in notice which hand is the first to become lifted. For westerners, the left hand is the first to rise. This is called chest breathing. For this exercise, it will be important for the right hand to lift up first. So now we will begin.

3. Take a slow, deep breath into your stomach. Be sure that your right hand is the first to be lifted up. Count to four as you breathe in. Hold the breath in your stomach for a count of four.

4. Slowly exhale that breath counting to four and see that your right hand in returning to its beginning position. Hold your lungs empty of air for a count of four.

5. Begin the process again by breathing in for a count of four, holding for a count of four, exhaling for a count of four, and remaining empty for a count of four. Do this for five minutes if you can.

NOTE: If you find that this breathing exercise is very easy for you, then you can increase the number to 6, 8, 10, etc. An ultimate number would be 20 or more.

While performing this breathing exercise, become aware of how your body is responding to the breath. Does your body feel like it is struggling with the breath? Do you feel resistance or pain? Do you sense a color, or form to the breath?

If you had to describe the breath, would be white, light and free flowing? Or would it be dark and heavy? Observe how your mind or emotions are responding to the movements of your body and the breath. Are you feeling happiness or joy? Are you feeling depressed or sad?

How we bring the breath into our body can affect the way we nurture and nourish our body. Slow deep breaths of joy will bring much more oxygen into the organs than short breaths of frustration. What kind of breath and emotion do you want to feed your body?

Contracting the Hui-Yin Point

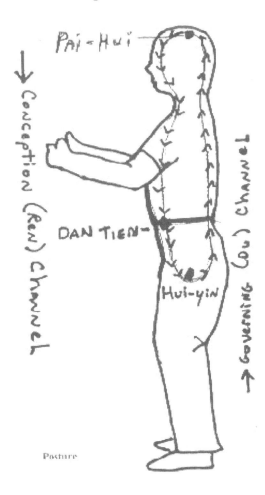

Another way to increase the intensity and flow of the breath is to contract the Hui-yin point while you are breathing. This is a common practice among yogis. The Hui-yin point is located between the genitals and the anus. This point is also called the Perineum Point. For women, contracting this point is much like doing a Kegel exercise. This point also represents an energy gateway where energy can either be stored or released.

To Do:
1. Place the tip of your tongue on the roof of your mouth just behind your front teeth and contract your Hui-Yin point.
2. Take a slow, deep breath in. See the energy coming into your nose as you inhale and run down the front of your body to the Hui-Yin point.
3. At the Hui-Yin point, you will exhale the breath up your spine seeing the energy flowing up your back and into your head.
4. When you are ready to release this breath, you can breathe this breath unto your client in areas of need, such as stagnate energy spots, closed chakras, releasing emotions, debris in aura, and much, much more.

Chapter Three
The Practice of Makko Ho

The Makko Ho exercises should be practiced once a day to ensure the benefits of a regular routine. The best of time of day to practice your Makko Ho exercises would be upon waking in the morning. By practicing the exercises in the morning, it will help your body to ease out of its stiffness as it gently awakens.

When the Makko Ho exercises are done slowly in the evening, the exercises may refresh the body and mind and can even enhance the sleep of the exerciser because it tends to release the tensions and stress of the day. But for some, doing any form of exercises in the evening may lead to a sleepless night as exercise, and even breath work, tends to increase the circulation and energy levels of the practitioner. So decide for yourself which is right for you and do it!

Makko Ho exercises will help to disperse areas in the body where Qi has become blocked or stagnant. By increasing the flow of energy to these afflicted areas, you can help to nurture that area and rebalance your body.

As a side note, whenever one area of the body is suffering due to the lack of the natural flow of energy to it, the body as a whole suffers. When we bring back the natural flow of energy to the body, we help to balance the body as a whole by replenishing the cells, organs and tissues.

It is recommended that the entire sequence of exercises should be carried out three times a day. It is also suggested that the exercises be performed in a general order, or sequence, as listed below.

The sequence is as follows:

Bladder and Kidneys - Water

Triple Heater and Heart Protector - Fire

Lungs and Large Intestine - Metal

Heart and Small Intestine - Fire

Liver and Gall Bladder - Wood

Spleen and Stomach - Earth

To Do:

1. Do the following six exercises in the order given.

2. Take your time and breathe through each exercise. Allow yourself to focus on each of the exercises as you are performing them.

3. Visualize the element of the exercise that you are working on.

4. Perform each individual exercise three times before moving on to the next one.

5. Repeat the entire sequence of six exercises and notice which of the exercises came easy to you and which exercise was painful.

6. Choose the exercise you liked the best and do it slowly feeling nurtured by it.

7. Choose the exercise you liked the least and do it more quickly. Repeat the exercise until you are able to release the tension or emotion that is attached to it, or until you begin to feel tired. Most people dislike an exercise because the energy is blocked or stagnant in that meridian. Instead of ignoring it, you are working to disperse that blockage or stagnation which will ultimately make you feel better when you are successful.

8. Repeat the whole sequence of exercises one more time and note any changes in yourself, your body, your mind, and in your sensations as you move.

9. Rest on the floor for a few minutes and allow yourself time to assimilate and relax.

10. Use the breathing technique given, or use one of your own.

Chapter Four
The Organ Systems and the Meridian Pairing

The Large Intestine and the Lung Meridians

The Large Intestine Meridian

The Large Intestine is associated with the skin, arm problems and nasal obstructions. The lung meridian deals with breathing and stiffness. It is also responsible for the elimination of waste products our bodies. It is through the large intestine that the food we eat and the water we drink get filtered out, the essential vitamins and minerals are sent on to the small intestines where they can be absorbed into our bodies to provide vital energy and thanks to the large intestine, the waste matter is taken on out of the digestive tract. If waste matter gets stuck here, the stagnation usually results in constipation, etc. This is why we can look at the Large Intestine as the ability to "Let Go".

The Large Intestine is an integral part of the digestive system. Along with the small intestine, the large intestine helps with the digesting and eliminating of waste products from our bodies. The Large Intestine looks like pink coils of muscle that stretch 5 feet long. The Small Intestine, regardless of its name, is actually longer than the Large Intestine-an amazing 20 feet. It is the not the length that gives the Intestines their name, it is their diameter. The Large Intestine is wider than the Small Intestine.

The Large Intestine is located just below the Small Intestine. The Large Intestine takes the indigestible parts of the food and absorbs the liquid from it. After the liquid has been absorbed, the semisolid waste product, or feces, it formed. The feces is then pushed down through the Large Intestine into the rectum for evacuation.

Some people believe that the state of the health and well-being for the body lies in its proper elimination. Some proponents to colon cleansings believe that you should be able to evacuate after every meal, that's three times a day, to insure a proper homeostasis within the body. Constipation is the lack of elimination for one or more days.

Most women have problems with the colon due to the female hormones estrogen and progesterone. These hormones have been known to relax the colon muscles. It is the colon that halts the movements of stools by contractions. When this muscle is relaxed, you may get diarrhea. So women should realize that this is a standard problem during "that time of the month". This usually occurs during the first two days on the menses and may also happen right before the menses. Doctors may prescribe over the counter anti diarrhea drugs containing loperamide hydrochloride such as Imodium A-D, but I just say, ride it out. Eat more fiber. It will last only a few days.

The Large Intestine is associated with the following:

Shoulder Joint pains

Nasal obstruction

Runny nose

Fever

Facial Tension

Diarrhea

Rash

Toothache

Sore legs

Any Arm problem (including pain and fatigue)

Elimination

Element is Water Large

Intestine is Yang

Deals with the skin Sense

is Smell Taste is Spicy

Sound is crying

Emotion is Melancholy

The Large Intestine helps the functioning of the lungs

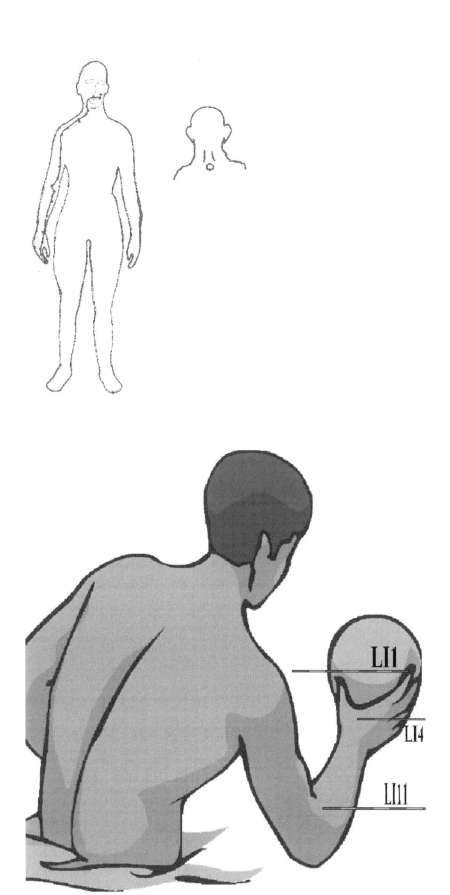

The Lung Meridian

The Lungs are in charge of the inhaling and exhaling of air. This air is vital to our existence as the air brings in oxygen to the blood. This oxygen is used to feed and nourish the cells of our body. When we take in too little air, the cells begin to starve and die. They can no longer reproduce themselves as they should and the body begins to age. With a depleted supply of oxygen, the organs begin to denigrate. They are not receiving the oxygen they need to do the functions within the body they created to do. The exhalations are used to release out of the body, stagnate air and particles of toxins from the lungs. This keeps the lungs in a healthier state of being.

The lungs are about the size of two footballs and are located in your chest. They are made of elastic tissue and filed with interlacing networks of tubes and sacs. This network of tubes and sacs carry air while the blood vessels carry the blood. The lungs not only supply oxygen to the body, it also disposes of carbon dioxide, filters and stores the blood, and defends the body against all outside invading agents of infection. Believe it or not, you take in an average of 20,000 breaths a day. So remember, breathe-and breathe deeply-you are feeding the very cells of your body!

Many Americans suffer from problems of the lungs, among them are cancer, allergies, and asthma. The world is filled with pollens and other breathing irritants such as strong perfumes, newsprint, pets, dust, etc.

What can you do?

If dust is your problem, consider a special filtered vacuum cleaner. If you are allergic to the cat, get rid of the cat. Since rugs foster mites and pollens, get rid of the carpets. Since humidity feeds pollens, keep your home as dry as possible. To help your odds of avoiding lung cancer, you can do the following: Don't smoke. If you do smoke, quit Eat fruits and vegetables (They contain beta-carotene which fight off free radicals).

Check for radon. (Radon is more common in the northern states where homes have been built over abandoned coal mines). This gas has been attributed to 16,000 lung cancer deaths a year. Six out of every 1,000 American women are expected to get emphysema in this country.

Although there is nothing you can do to reverse the damaged lung tissue, if you are one of these women, aside from quitting smoking, here are some things you can do you improve your life: Exercise. Exercise the arm and shoulder muscles to help with shortness of breath Take Vitamin C (recommended dose is 250 milligrams twice a day) Take Vitamin E (recommended dose is 800 units twice a day)

Practice pursed lip breathing. You pucker your lips up like you are going to whistle, then breathe in through your nose and out through your pursed lips. Do this for 5 to 10 minutes. Repeat this breathing exercise for 2 to 3 times a day.

* Note: Vitamin C and Vitamin E can be toxic at high levels. Please check with your doctor before taking additional dosages of Vitamins or Minerals.

The Lung Meridian deals with the following:

Sore throat, cough, colds

Painful breathing, congestion, headaches, asthma

Bell's palsy

Elbow pain, stiffness

Elimination

Element is metal

Emotion is melancholy

Lungs are yin

Deals with the skin

Sense is smell

Taste is spicy

Sound is crying

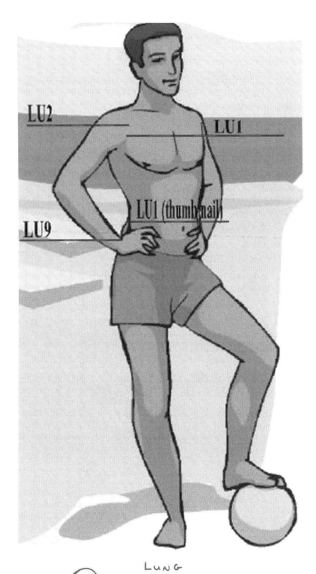

LUNG

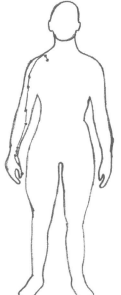

Makko Ho Exercise #1

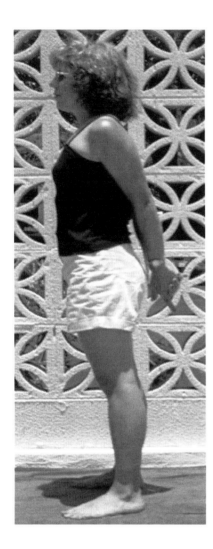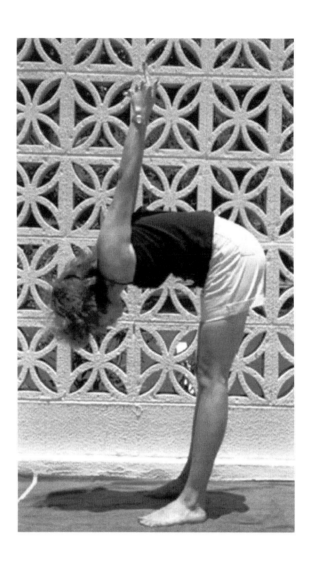

To Do:

Stand with your feet shoulder width apart. Link your thumbs behind your back. (**Note:** if you cannot clasp your hands together behind your back, then use a towel and grab it on each end.) Breathe in, fill your body and lungs with oxygen as you straighten your arms and open up your chest. As you exhale, bend slowly forward while keeping your back, arms and legs straight. Hold this bent over position for three sets of breaths* and return to the starting position. Repeat two more times for a total of three sets of this exercise.

* A set is one inhalation and one exhalation. A set of three breaths would be three inhalations in and three exhalations out.

NOTE: Very few people can raise their arms behind their back as the picture indicates. Do **NOT** force your arms into this position. You can only do the best you can in that direction - nothing more.

Note of caution - if you generally experience dizziness or become light headed with bending forward, please omit this exercise.

Another option would be to place a chair in front of you and hold on to the chair for support or sit in a chair or on the end of your bed and perform the exercise to the best of your ability. Be safe - not sorry!

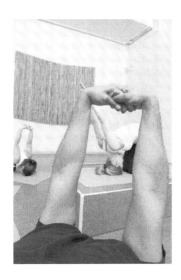

Wrist Stretch

To Do:

Stand or sit and bring your hands behind your back. Interlace your fingers if you can. Breathe in, fill your body and lungs with oxygen as you straighten your arms and open up your chest. As you exhale, bend slowly forward while keeping your back, arms and legs straight. Hold this bent over position for three sets of breaths* and return to the starting position. Repeat two more times for a total of three sets.

Many meridians begin or end at the fingers and toes. In stretching out the wrists, we are activating many of the meridian systems allowing for a free flow of energy to occur.

Exercise Option: If you cannot bring your arms behind your back, then bring them out in front of you and perform the same exercise in the front of your body. You will still be able to gain vital benefits in performing this exercise.

Another way to accomplish the above exercise if you have trouble standing is follow the picture below:

Makko Ho Exercise #1 Alternate(A)

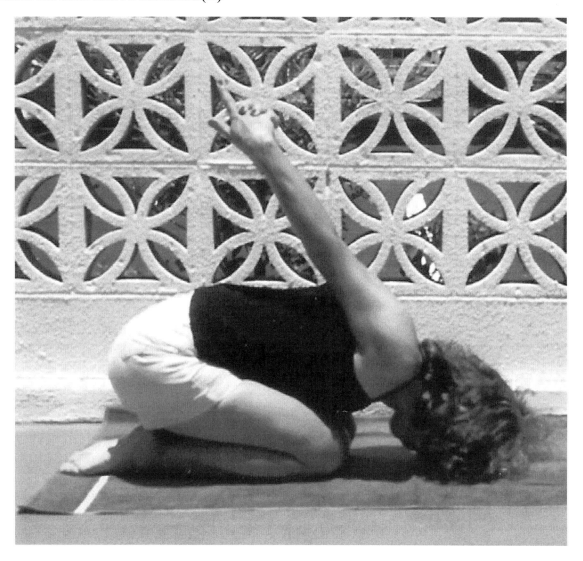

To Do:

Kneel on the floor. (If you find it difficult to kneel on the floor on your knees, you might want to try to place a pillow under your buttocks to take the stress off your knees.) Interlace your fingers behind your back, extending your index fingers. Straighten your arms.

Inhale. As you exhale bend your body forward as far as you can. If you want to, you can rest your forehead on the ground in front of you. Do three breath sets while in this position. On the third exhalation, return to your starting position. Repeat this exercise for a total of three repetitions.

Makko Ho Exercise #1 Alternate(B)-Using a Stretch Band or Towel

If you cannot clasp your hands together, or if you have shoulder problems, then you will need to try something else. You can use a belt, stretch band, or even a towel and perform the same exercise for the same benefits.

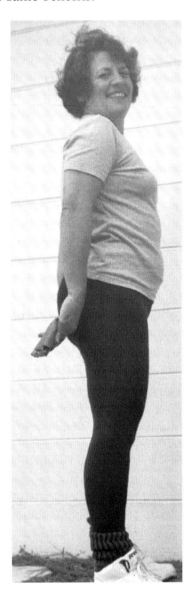

Adding the Element of Metal

Metal concerns itself with the exchange of air and breathing. It is also concerned with elimination, of letting go. Constipation is caused by our need to hold on, not to let go. So for this exercise, we will concentrate on the taking in of breath (air) and releasing (letting go) of the breath.

Throughout the exercise become aware of your breath. As you breathe in, notice how easily you take the breath into your body. As you exhale, become aware of how the breath feels as it leaves your body. Be aware of your sensations and experiences throughout this movement.

Chapter Five
The Small Intestine and the Heart Meridians

The Small Intestine Meridian
        The Small Intestine Meridian deals with quality of the blood and the Heart Meridian deals with the blood vessels.

        It is in the Small Intestine that the food we eat and the water we drink are used to provide our body's with vital energy. The food is broken down in the small intestine and separated and absorbed into the body. The Small Intestine affects the quality of our blood and our tissues. A healthy Small Intestine means a healthy blood quality.

        The Small Intestine is part of the digestive system. Despite its name, the small intestine is actually longer than the Large Intestine. The Small Intestine is an amazing 20 feet long! The Small Intestine is not as wide as the Large Intestine, but can still get the job done.

        To keep your Intestines healthy and happy, it is advised to use moderation when eating fresh fruits and drinking fruit juices. These items are high is one type of sugar called, fructose. Sometimes, too much fructose can get digested and seep through to the small intestine and colon. Once there, fructose is fermented by the bacteria that live there. This can result in bloating, gas, and even diarrhea. (Yes, you are actually feeding these bacteria). Don't stop eating fruits, just limit their intake. If you had to choose, choose to eat a piece of fruit rather than drinking it, it is easier to digest that way.

        Another thing to realize and perhaps eliminate from our diets is sorbitol.
Large amounts of sorbitol can cause gas and diarrhea. Sorbitol is readily found in sugarless gums. One stick of sugarless gum can contain as much as 2 grams of sorbitol

        Our system can only handle about 5 grams before it begins to complain.
Everyone is different. If you are one of the lucky ones, your system may be able to ingest up to 50 grams of sorbitol before your intestines begin to act up.
        Sorbitol can also be found in candies, medications and I have even seen it in ice cream. Be aware of other sweeteners such as xylitol and mannitol which can affect your body in the same way.

        So, if you have been having problems of bloating and gas and have not figure out its source, read the labels of the food you have been ingesting-the problem may lie there.

        Another culprit is the use of antacids. While the antacid may bring immediate relief, it may actually cause problems later. Of course, this depends on factors such as how many times you take the antacid, dietary problems, etc.

        The problem with antacids is that they contain magnesium which pulls the water from the body into the intestines leaving you with loose stools or diarrhea. Antacids that contain aluminum can cause constipation.

The Small Intestine also deals with emotions such as anxiety, emotional excitement, trauma, and even shock. All of these can affect the small intestine in an adverse way. It is best to practice emotional stability and add calmness to your life for a healthy small intestine.

Items associated with the Small Intestine are:

Ringing in the Ears
Shoulder pain
Neuralgia
Numbness/paralysis of the fingers

Element is Fire

Small Intestine is yang

Deals with blood vessels

Sense is speech

Taste is bitter

Sound is laughing

Emotion is joy

Spiritual awareness

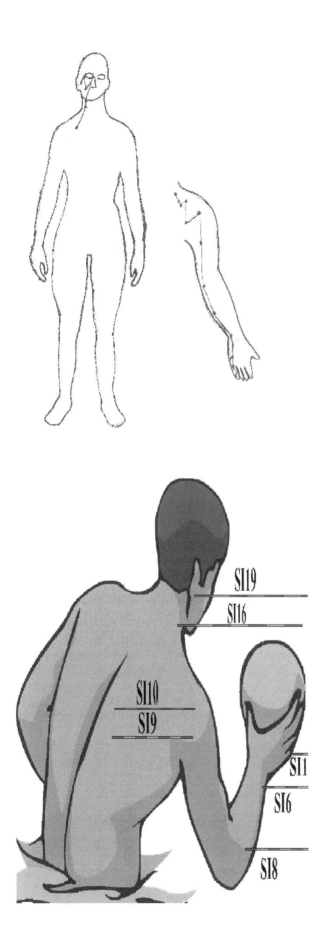

The Heart Meridian

The Heart governs the blood and blood vessels. It pumps the vital blood to all areas of our body. It replenishes and feeds every organ and tissue in our body. A healthy heart means healthy organs and tissues.

The Heart is about the size of man's fist and weighs just ten ounces. The heart pumps an amazing 2,000 gallons of blood through 60,000 miles of blood vessels every day. Your heart beats an average of 100,000 times each and every day. Through health habits, you can expect your heart to last through 2.5 billion contractions over your lifetime.

Our worse fears are heart attacks and strokes. These cardiovascular problems are caused when the heart or the blood vessels get clogged. These arteries get clogged with fat deposits, called plaque. This plaque continues to build up until it impedes the flow of blood through the blood vessels.

Arteries can also grow stiff with age or damaged by disease. Each year 300,000 Americans suffer from a heart attack. Of that number, 30,000 can expect to die from that attack within 3 days. Heart disease is something you can help to prevent through simple exercise and proper dietary adjustments.

The Heart houses the mind and our emotions. Emotions such as Joy are good for the heart and help it to stay healthy and strong.

Avoid anger, resentments, revenge, etc. It can "eat up" your joy and damage the functioning of your heart. Think about that as you do the following exercise. If there is something that is "eating" away at you, now is a good time to learn to release it and let it go. Take charge of your own health and well-being.

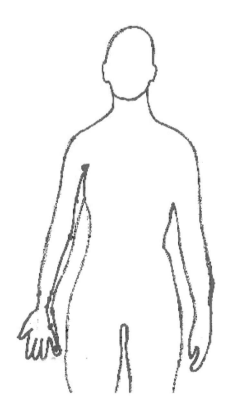

The Heart Meridian deals with:

Insomnia

Irritability

Constipation

Heart palpitations

Reviving an unconscious patient

Heart problems

Element is fire

Heart is yin

Deals with the blood vessel

Sense is speech

Taste is bitter

Sound is laughing

Emotion is joy

Spiritual awareness

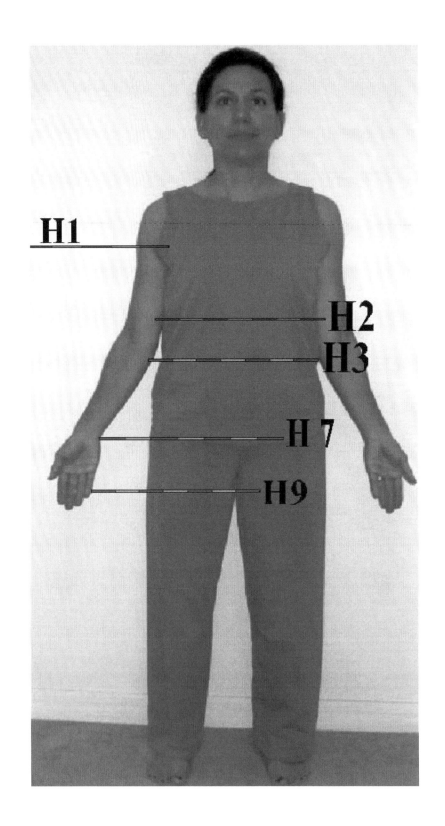

Makko Ho Exercise #2

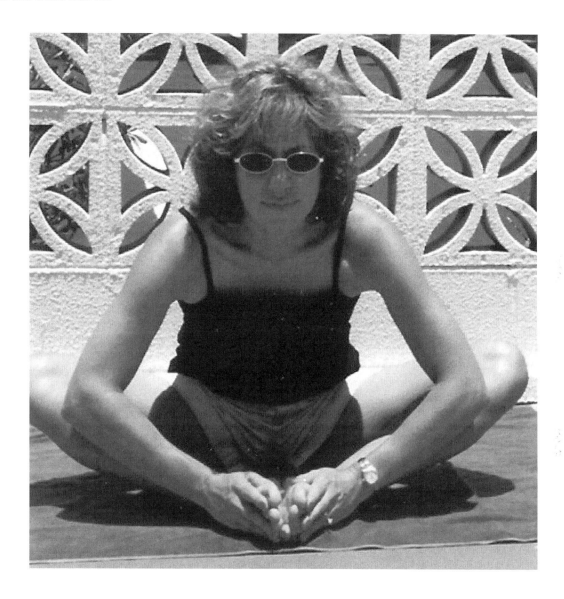

To Do:

Sit on the floor and place the soles of your feet together. Draw the heels of your feet close to your body and place your right elbow on the inside of your right knee and your left elbow on the inside of your left knee. Breathe in.

As you exhale, draw your body down bending your elbows and easing your knees to the floor. (Please note that 99 out of 100 people with NOT be able to touch their knees to the floor, so don't force the movement, just ease in the general direction of the floor).

Hold this position for three sets of breath. Feel the expansion in your back. On the third exhaled breath, return to starting position. Repeat for two more sets.

Visualizing the Element of Fire

For this exercise, we add the element of fire. This fire brings joy and warmth into our lives. This fire is also involved in food assimilation as well as emotions in our body.

When you think of this type of fire involved in food, what comes to mind?

A flame from a gas stove, or barbecue pit?

Do you imagine the flame from a pizza oven or boiler room?

How about an electric blanket?

Whatever image comes to mind is the right image for you. Fire increases the temperature of your body and in so doing increases the circulation in your body giving you warmth. So, during this exercise, hold an image of fire in your mind. Breathe in the fire of joy and warmth Exhale emotions such as anger, envy, etc.

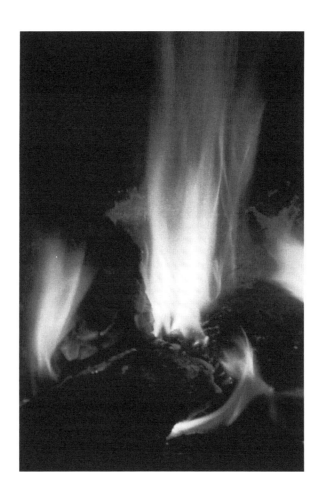

Chapter Six
The Bladder and Kidney Meridians

The Bladder Meridian

The Bladder Meridian is charge of purification and the Kidneys are in charge of storing Qi. The Bladder is in charge of the storing of any overflow and fluid secretions in the body. It helps to regulate the body. The Bladder offers us the courage and ability to move forward in our lives.

The Bladder Meridian is associated with the following:

Easy labor
Sciatica, tired legs, muscle spasms
Dizziness, epilepsy, nausea,
Bed-wetting,
Small/Large intestines
Sexual strength
Lower back pain, poor circulation, weak heart, exhaustion, irritability
Sweating, fevers
Asthma, breathing problems in general
Poor or tired vision, swollen eyes
Constipation
PMS, menstrual irregularities
Problems of the Stomach, Spleen, Liver and Kidneys
Vomiting, Nausea, and Hiccups

Element is water

Bladder is yang

Deals with the bones

Sense is hearing

Taste is salty

Sound is groaning

Emotion is fear

Associated with ambition and willpower

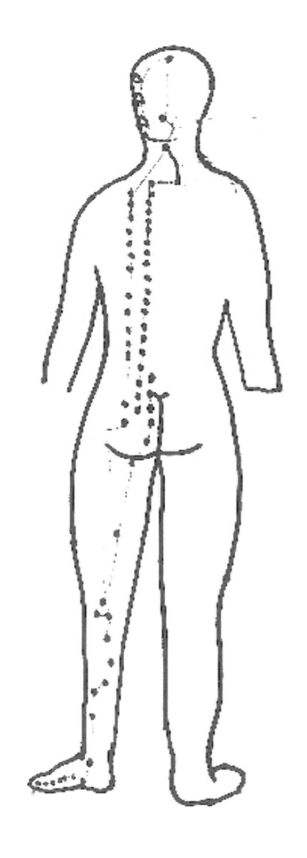

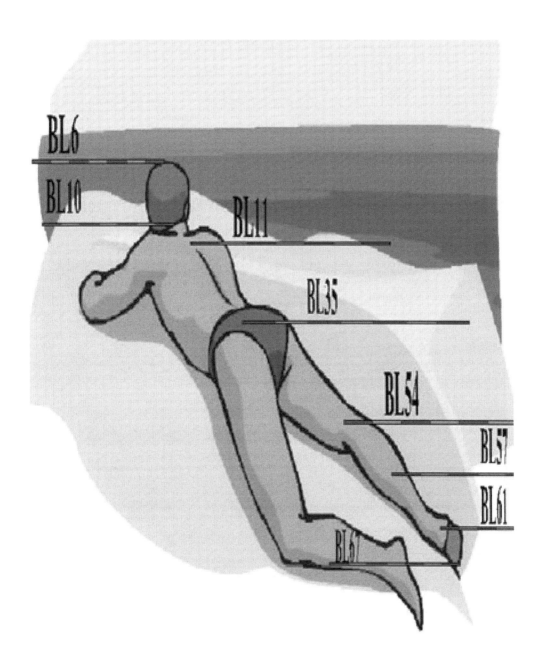

The Kidney Meridian

The Kidney Meridian is used to store fundamental "Qi" in the body until other organs need it. The Kidney Meridian also governs birth, growth, reproduction and development. It also nourishes and supports the spine, the bones, and the brain. The Kidneys offer vitality, direction and will-power. It is also associated with ambition.

The Kidney Meridian is associated with the following:

Kidney malfuctions

Epilepsy

Dizziness

Menstrual pain

Revival

Element is water

Kidney is yin

Deals with the bones

Sense is hearing

Taste is salty

Sound is groaning

Emotion is fear

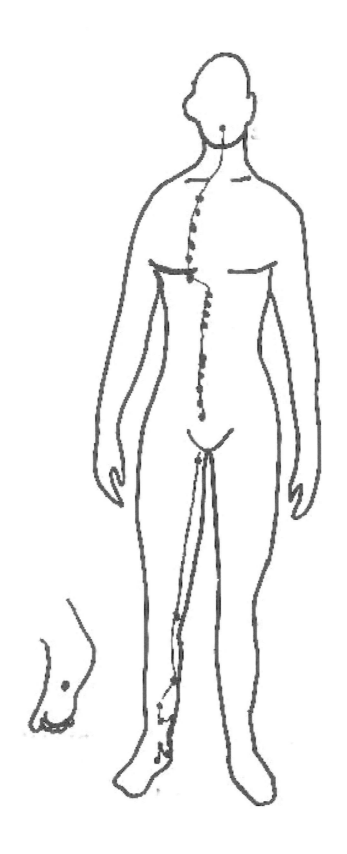

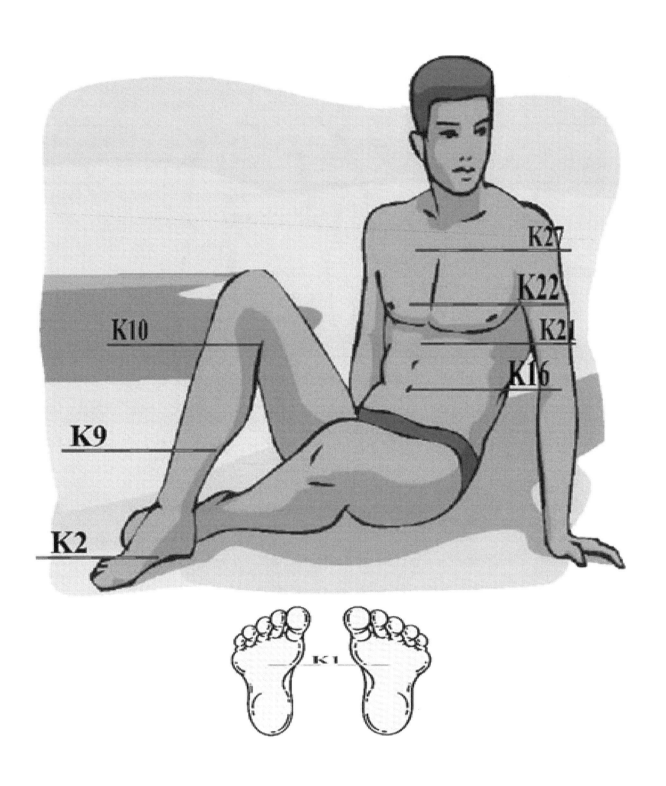

Makko Ho Exercise #3

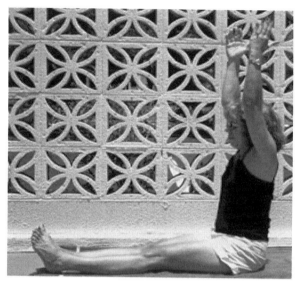 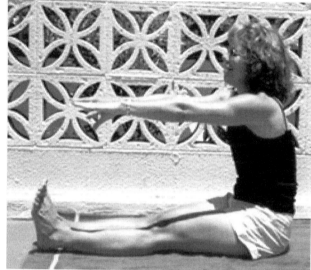

To Do:

Sit upright on the floor with your legs out in front of you in a parallel position. Your hips are wide apart and your toes are pointing upward at a 90 degree angle.
Inhale and draw your arms up above your head with your palms facing each other. Keep your back straight.

As you exhale, ease your upper torso forward, bending from the hips with your arms reaching forwards and parallel to the legs (Note: you are NOT aiming downward toward your toes, but forward at least a foot above your toes.) Look ahead.

Hold this position while you perform three sets of breath, with each breath you are trying to ease forward a little bit more.

On the third exhaled breath, you return to your starting position. Do this exercise for three sets all together.

Adding the Element of Water

You can now add the visualization of water to this exercise. Water represents fluidity. So during this exercise you will visualization the fluidity and ease flow of breath throughout your body. Water releases fear from your mind and body. Remember how tense we become when frightened and fearful?

When you imagine water, what comes to your mind?

Do you imagine a lake, river, or stream?

Do your thoughts flow like a waterfall?

Whatever represents water to you is what you will visualize while performing this exercise.

Become the water, pure and easy-flowing.

Inhale the easy flowing water

Exhale away tension, fear, and stress.

Feel the water clean your body and make it new and whole again.

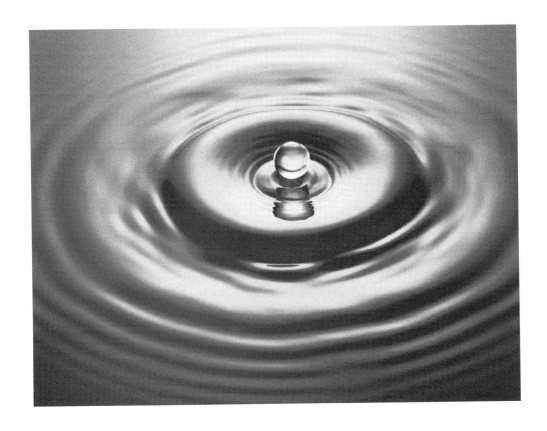

Chapter Seven
The Triple Heater and Heart Protector Meridians

The Triple Heater Meridian

The Triple Heater is also known as the Triple Warmer. The Triple Heater is responsible for the transportation of energy, blood and heat to the peripheral parts of the body (like the hands and feet).

The Triple Heater is associated with the emotion of being helpful and emotionally interactive.

The Triple Heater Meridian deals with:

Shoulder joint pain

Blood vessels

Element is Fire

Triple Heater is yang

Sense is speech

Taste is bitter

Sound is laughing

Emotion is joy

Spiritual awareness

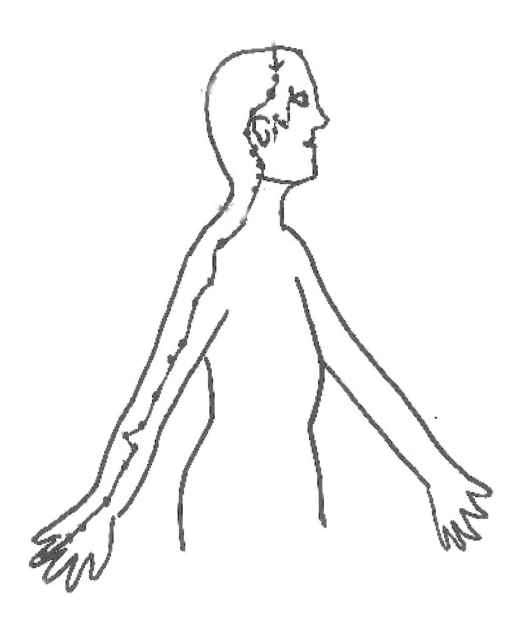

Heart Protector Meridian

The Heart Protector is also known as the Heart Governor. The official job of the Heart Protector is to protect the heart and closely related emotional responses. It is related to the central circulation. The Heart Protector influences relationships with others.

The Heart Protector (or Heart Constrictor) Meridian deals with the following:

Exhaustion

Nausea

Vomiting

Insomnia

Palpitations

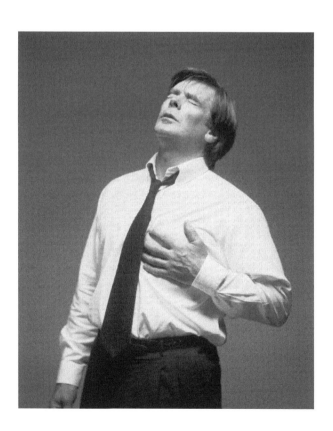

Makko Ho Exercise #4

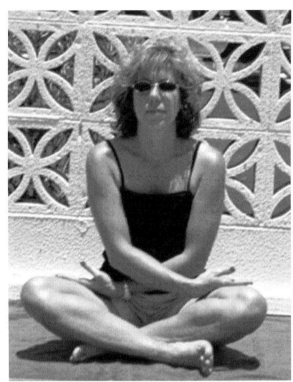 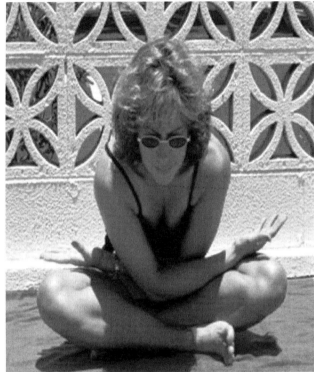

To Do:
Sit on the floor in a cross-legged position. (The above illustration is a simple version of the harder to do lotus position). Cross your arms and rest your hands on your thighs with the palms facing upwards and your fingers together. Breathe in.

As you exhale, slide your hands out sideways away from your body. Keep the palms of the hands flat and horizontal. Bring your body forward. Hold this position for a set of three breaths and on the third exhaled breath return to starting position. Repeat this exercise for two more sets for a total of three sets.

Adding Visualization

Fire affects the function of the body on the physical level. Fire deals with our immunity and our ability to cope with stress. As you perform this exercise, think of the element of fire. You can visualization a gentle candle glowing, a fire in the fireplace, or even a bonfire in the middle of a football field. When you think of fire, what comes to your mind? Use that as your visualization for this exercise. Become the fire. As you inhale, you inhale the heat of the fire and send it throughout your body to warm and strengthen. As you exhale, you release the pent up heat (anger) of your body.

Chapter Eight
The Gall Bladder and Liver Meridians

The Gall Bladder

The Gall Bladder is responsible for the storing of bile by the liver. The Gall Bladder then distributes the bile to the small intestine. The Gall Bladder is for making practical applications of ideas and decision-making. Both the Gall-Bladder and Liver Meridians deal with the muscles of the body.

The Gall Bladder meridian is associated with the following:

Eye problems
Headaches
Dizziness
Ringing in the ears
Common cold symptoms
Shoulder pain
Lack of milk in nursing mothers
Gall Bladder ailments, stomach aches, menstrual pain, or PMS
Digestive problems. vomiting
Sciatica, lower back aches
Circulation in legs, tired legs, varicose veins
Ankle, leg or foot pain

Element is wood

Gall Bladder is yang

Sense is sight

Taste is sour

Contains much anger and shouting

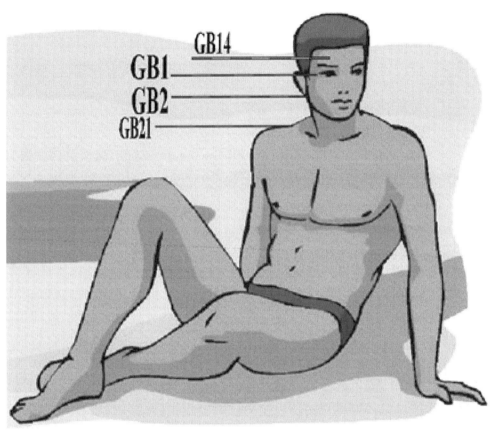
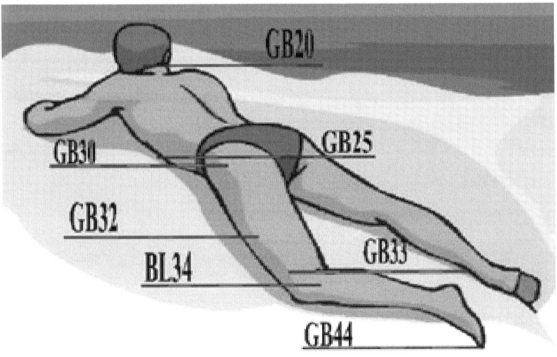

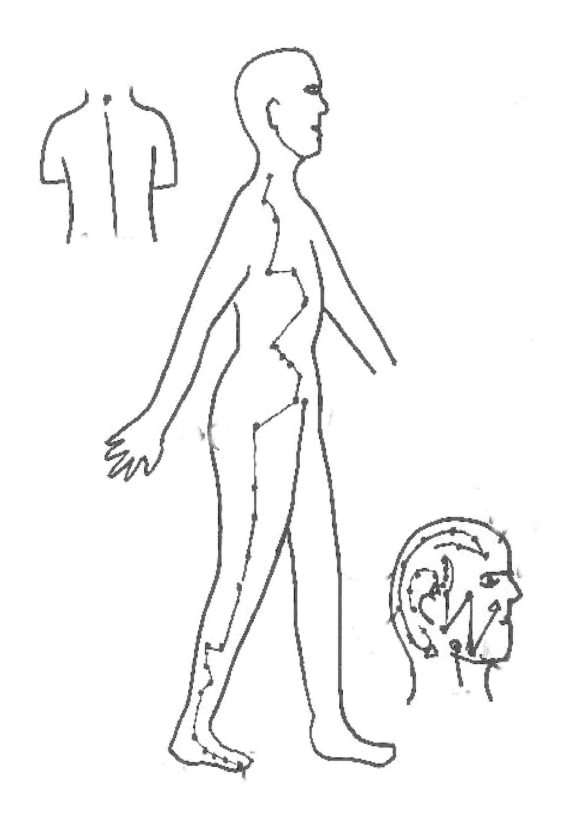

The Liver Meridian

The Liver Stores the blood to be used throughout the body. The liver ensures the free flow of Qi throughout the body. The liver is creative and full of ideas.

The Liver Meridian deals with the following:

Headaches

Dizziness

Arthritis in the ankle

PMS, menstrual cramps

Frigidity

Abdominal pains, vomiting

Lower Back, or rib aches and pains

Poor lactation in nursing mothers

Element is wood

Liver is yin

Deals with the muscles

Sense is sight

Taste is sour

Contains much anger and shouting

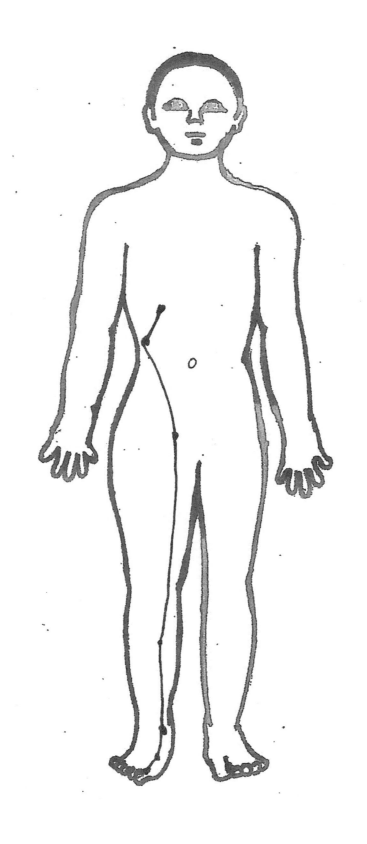

Liver Meridian

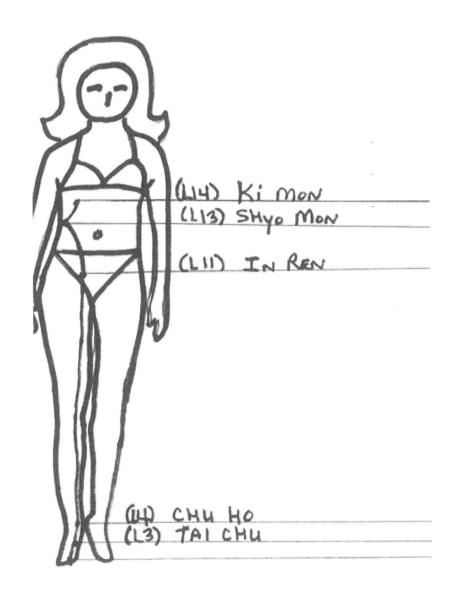

Makko Ho Exercise #5

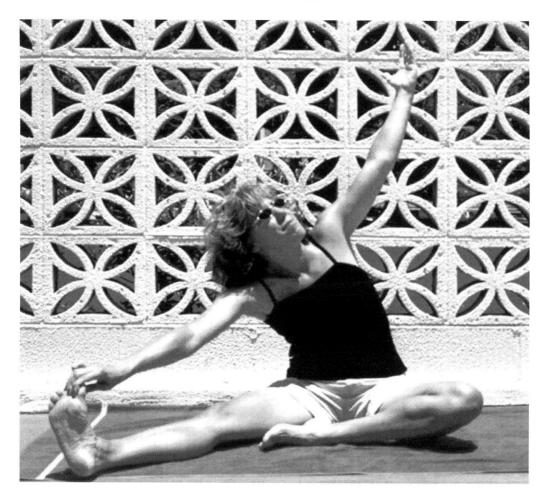

To Do:

Sit upright on the floor with your right leg extended and the toes of your right leg pointed upwards. Bend your left leg with your left foot touching the inside of your right leg. Grab your right toe with your right hand (If you cannot reach your right toe, then grab your ankle, calf, or knee). Inhale and raise your left arm up towards the ceiling, looking up at your hand.

As you exhale, lean sideways towards the right to with your body and left arm extended over your head reaching for your right toe. Do NOT force this move and do NOT allow your body to collapse. Do NOT strain. Look upwards. Keep your chest open. Hold this position for three sets of breaths.

On the third exhaled breath return to starting position. Repeat this whole process for a total of three sets. When finished, extend your left leg and bend your right leg. Repeat the same process on the other side of your body for a total of three sets on the left

Adding the Element of Wood

While doing this exercise, you will add the element of wood. Concentrate on the qualities of your favorite tree or the properties of wood that you associate with. In particular, concentrate on the strength and flexibility of a tree when it is in a state of health. Explore these qualities in your own body. Feel strength within your own spine. Your spine supports you throughout the day and yet feel how flexible the spine can be as it allows you to bend forward and backward, and from side to side. The spine is strong and yet flexible. That is how you should be.

Picture in your mind your favorite tree. See it clearly in your minds' eye. What color is your favorite tree? How does it make you feel?

How tall is your favorite tree?

See you become your favorite tree. Are you tall and strong?

Are you welcoming? Inviting?

Do you allow yourself to stand rigid against new ideas and new ways of doing things, or are you open and flexible to new ideas and thoughts?

Are you stubborn and rigid? Or do you go with the flow? Are you bendable, flexible?

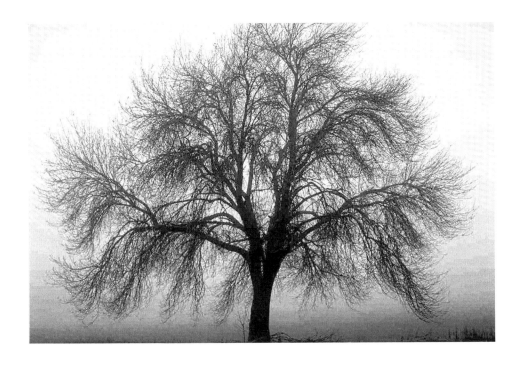

Chapter Nine
The Spleen and Stomach Meridians

The Spleen Meridian

The Spleen corresponds to the function of the pancreas in Westerns terms. The Spleen governs the general digestion including saliva and gastric bile. The Spleen is also responsible for the secretions from the small intestines. The Spleen also provides the reproductive hormones related to the breasts and ovaries. The Spleen is about 5 inches longs and purplish in color. It is located under the lower rib cage on the left side of the body.

The main job of the Spleen is to maintain the health of the flesh, the connective soft tissue and the muscle. It removes the iron from exhausted red blood cells and transports them to the bone marrow where the iron is reused in the making of hemoglobin (an oxygen bearing protein).

The Spleen also makes white blood cells and antibodies to fight bacteria and viruses. It filters out these intruders in our blood. Without the spleen, the liver and bone marrow would have to take up the fight, but nothing does as well as the spleen in fighting certain bacterial infections. The Spleen corresponds with our own self-image. Here is where our self-confidence and the desire to help others lie.

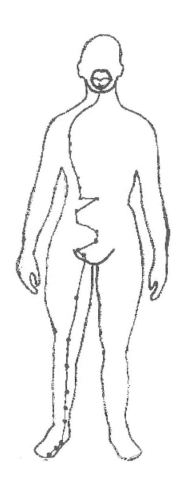

The Spleen Meridian deals with the following:

Knee pains

Itching

Hives

PMS

Menstrual pain

Spleen problems

Stomach problems

Element is earth

Spleen is yin

Deals with the flesh

Sense is taste

Taste is sweet

Sound is singing

Emotion is compassion

Deals with ideas and opinions

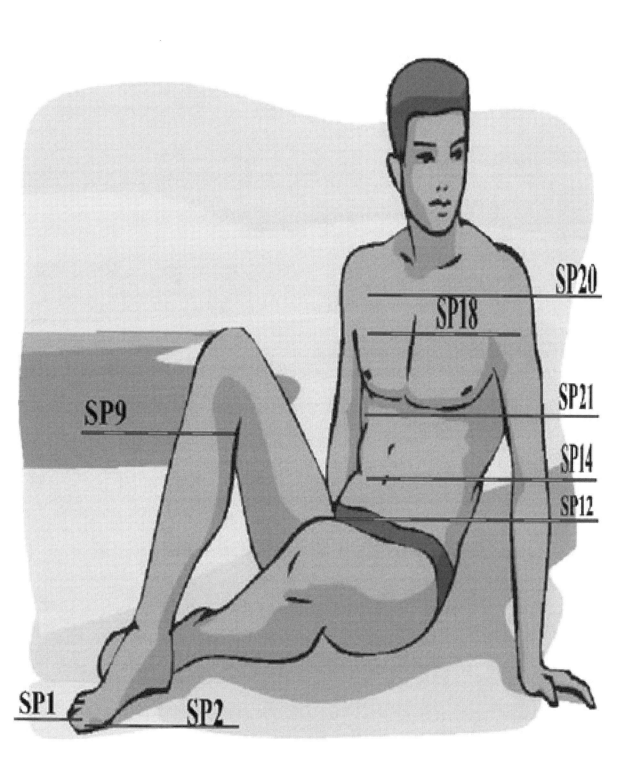

The Stomach Meridian

The Stomach is responsible for receiving the food we eat and the water we drink. It is here in the stomach, that this food and water is received and processed. The stomach is a J-shaped, balloon like sac that sits between the esophagus and the small intestine. It is about the size of a one-liter bottle when empty, and the size of a Thanksgiving dinner when full.

The stomach works through a series of expansions and contractions. It churns food out in contractions about every 20 seconds. In order to break down this food, the stomach uses gastric juices, like battery acid. In order to protect the stomach from the acid, the stomach lining produces a mucus. Food, alcohol, spicy or acidic foods, and even medications can increase the acid secretion and damage the stomach lining which can cause ulcers.

The medications most at fault for increasing stomach acids are the nonsteroidal anti-inflammatory drugs, also known as (NSAIDs). If you are unsure if the drugs you are taking belong to this family, read the label. If you need to take this medication, at least follow it with food and/or an antacid; don't take them on an empty stomach.

The Stomach is also the place where new ideas, thoughts, etc. are digested. Additional nourishment is here for mental and physical information. It provides a well-grounded, centered and reliable person. A person who has several bouts of indigestion, ulcers, or other stomach problems may be having trouble dealing with people, events, and/or situations that surround them. They may have trouble analyzing and digesting new ideas and concepts.

The Stomach meridian deals with all problems associated with the stomach.

Element is earth

Stomach is yang

Deals with the flesh

Sense is taste

Taste is sweet

Sound is singing

Emotion is compassion

Deals with ideas and opinions

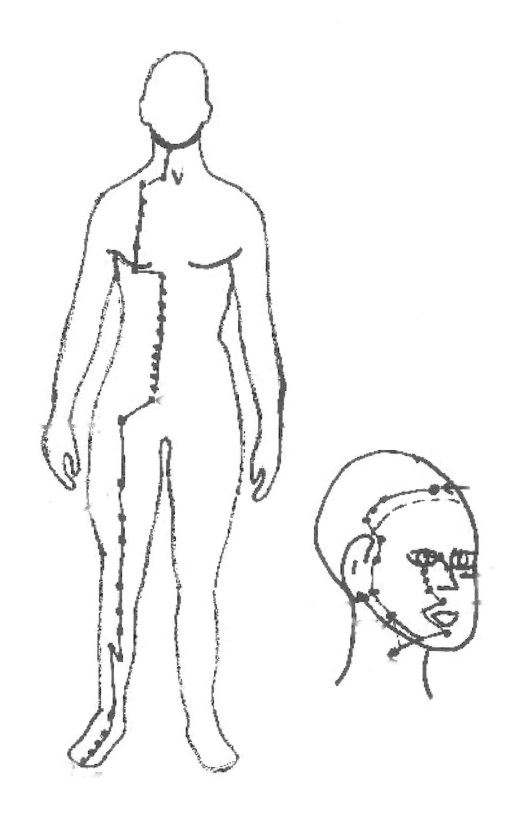

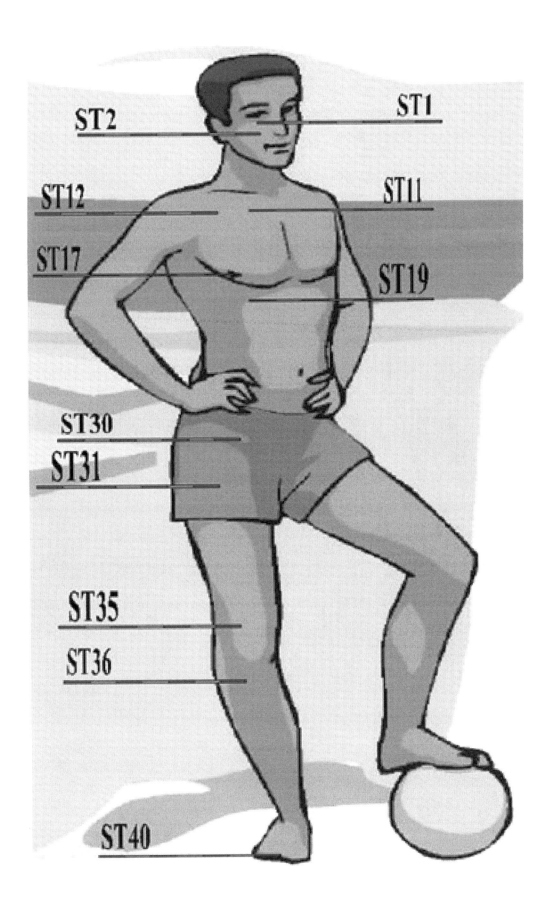

Makko Ho Exercise #6

Beginner Position #1

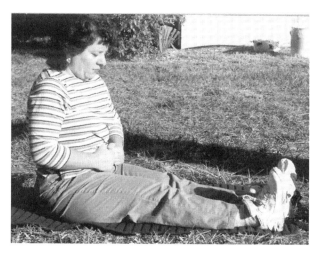 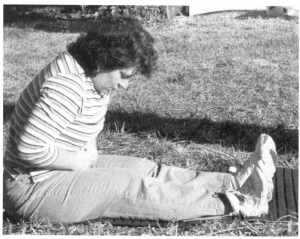

To Do:

Sit on the floor with your legs extended forward from your body.

Make your hands into two fists.

Place your two fists on your lower stomach area about 2-4" below the navel.

Breathe in.

As you exhale, lean your body forward. Hold this position for three sets of breath.

On the third exhalation, return to the starting position.

Repeat this process for two more sets for a total of three sets.

Position #2

(This exercise is for the more advanced student)

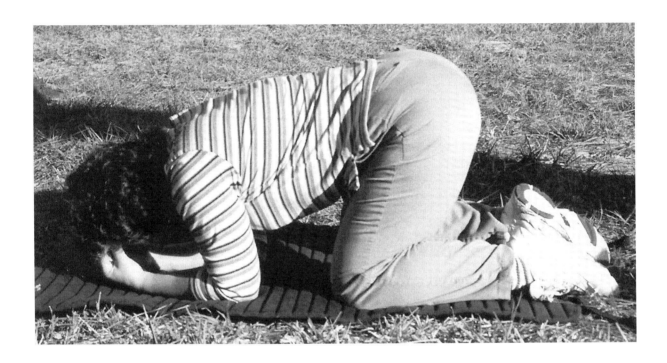

To Do:

Kneel on the floor and sit back on the heels of your feet. Tuck your toes in.

Place the fingertips of both of your hands on your face.

Breathe in.

As you exhale, bend forward until your head touches the floor.

Hold this position and breathe for three sets of breath.

On the third exhalation, return to the starting position.

Repeat the entire process for a total of three sets.

Adding the Element of Earth:
For this visualization you are part of the Earth. You are "Earth Mother" or "Earth Dad". See yourself as sympathetic, considerate and supportive. You care for those around you.

Now - Connect to the earth by trusting it.

Earth is the element of center and balance. Find yours. Become aware of your body alignment as you do these exercises. Do you easily fall forwards or backwards? Are you easily thrown "off balance"? If you said yes, then you must become aware of how your body moves and balances itself.

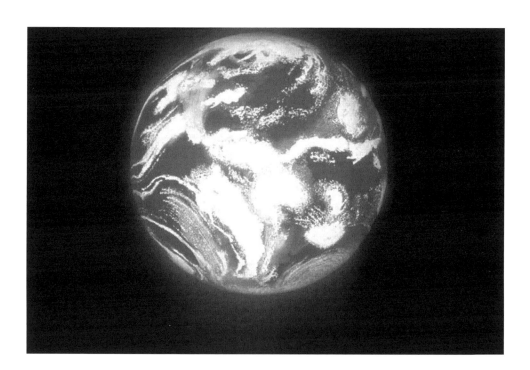

Additional exercise:

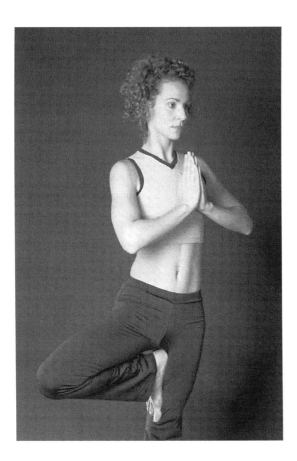
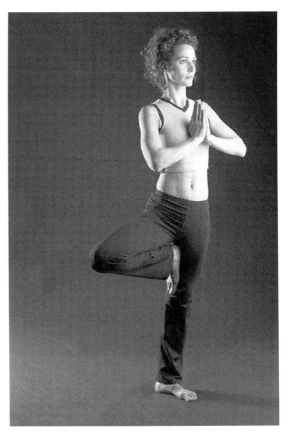

      Just stand nice and tall. Now, bend your right knee and lift your right foot off the ground. Stand here for a few minutes and become aware of your body begins to compensate for the shift in weight. Focus your thought and attention on what you are doing.

      Now, place the right foot back down on the ground and lift your left foot off the ground. Now that you are more focused and aware of what it is you are doing, did you find that your body needed less shifting and adjusting time? Good. Practice patience in the moment.

      For this visualization you are aware of all that is around you. You are very much in the moment. As you bend forward you are releasing stagnation and the past. Remember, you are living in the present now. Is there any hurt, worry, trauma or regrets you are keeping alive in the present? If there is, now is the time to release them into the past. You are here in the present now, release and let go as you exhale.

Chapter Ten

Finishing Exercises

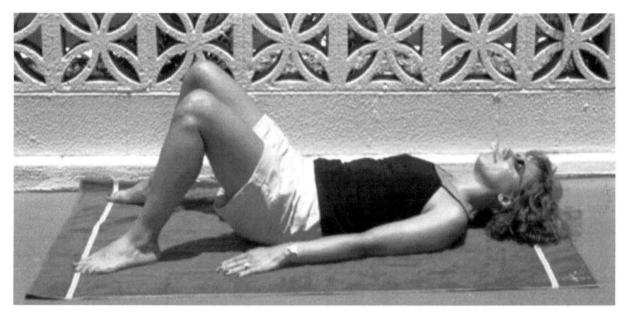

Note: If you suffer from lower back ache, please keep your knees bent during this exercise.

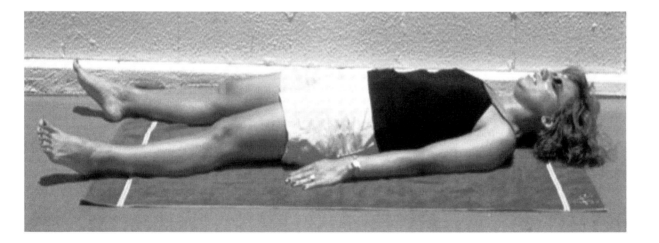

To Do:
After you have completed the whole sequence of exercises, lie flat on the floor with your eyes closed. Breathe gently in and out for a few minutes. Allow everything to settle in your body Bring your awareness to your body as a whole. How do you feel? Take an inventory of the areas of your body. Is there any tension? Is there any pain?

If you suffer from lower back aches, etc. choose the first position shown in the illustration. When you lie on the floor or any hard surface, bend your knees with your feet flat on the floor. If you wish, you can also use a rolled up towel placed under your knees for added comfort and back tension release.

Be comfortable. As you are lying on the floor, you may be aware of tingling sensations as your inner energy responds to your Makko Ho exercise session. Do not be alarmed. This is a good and welcomed thing. Breathe into your stomach and relax.

Take as much time as you need before ending this session and going about your day. Be aware of your resistances to these exercises, or any other forms of exercises. Do not become discouraged.

It will take at least two weeks of daily practice before you will feel the benefits of a Makko Ho program. The more time you devote to your practice - the greater and sooner the rewards. It is all up to you! If you are pressed for time, do 1 sequence of the exercises. This 1 sequence of 6 exercise movements will take less than 15 minutes.

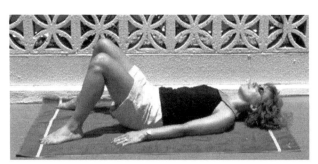 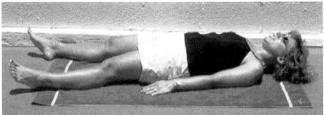

The Makko Ho Practice

Routine

Do the **complete sets of Makko Ho exercises** for three times in a consecutive sequence and finish the exercise program with the Finishing Exercise.

The sequence should be done in the following order:

Bladder and Kidney exercises

Triple Heart and Heart Protector exercises

Lungs and Large Intestine exercises

Heart and Small Intestine exercises

Liver and Gall-Bladder exercises

Spleen and Stomach exercises

NOTE: Do the above for a total of three sets and then add the following items listed below:

1. **When finished add:** Pick your least favorite exercise and repeat it for one set

2. **When finished add**: Pick your favorite exercise and repeat it for one set

3. **When finished add:** Finish off the exercise routine with the Finishing Exercise.

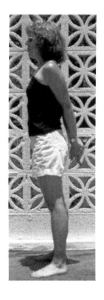 1a.
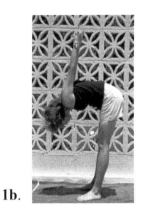 1b.
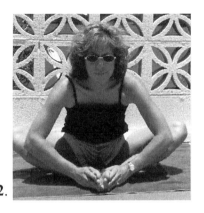 2.
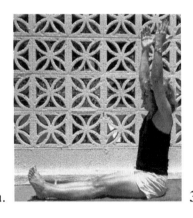 3a.
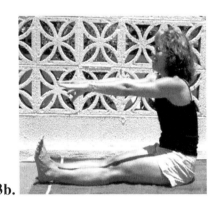 3b.
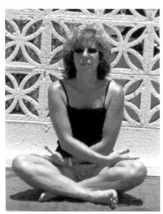 4a.
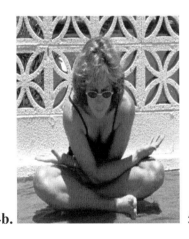 4b.
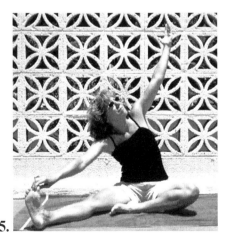 5.

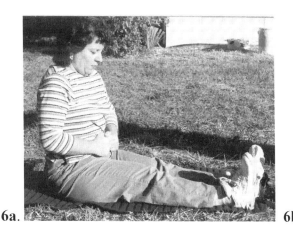
6a.
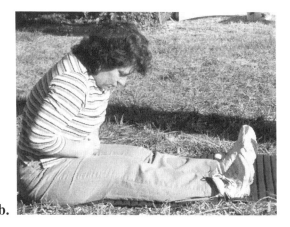
6b.

Finishing Exercises

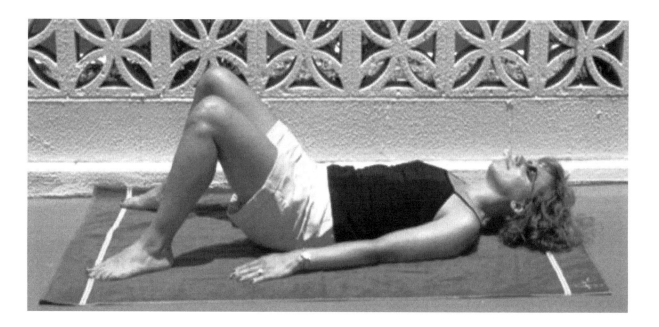

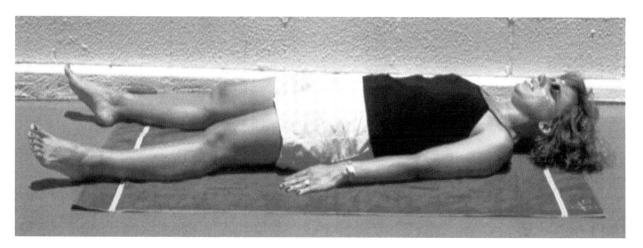

NOTES:

Chapter Eleven
The Old Food Guide Pyramid 2005

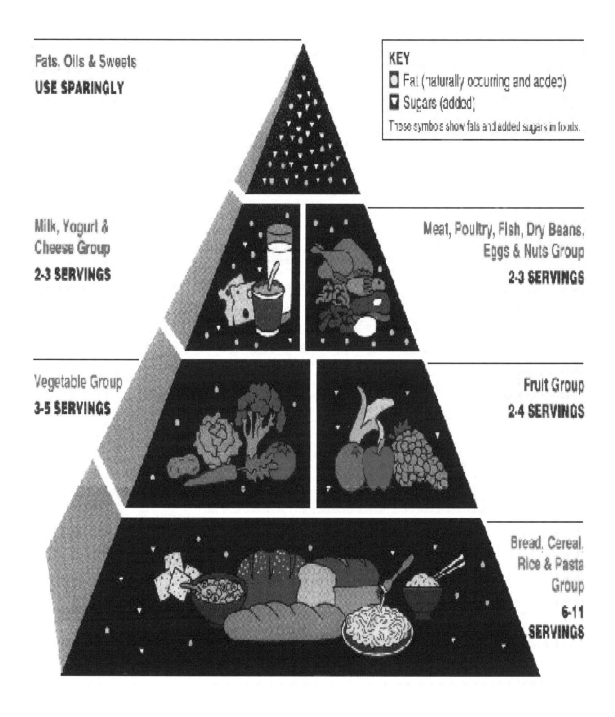

The Food Guide Pyramid on the previous page was developed by the U.S. Department of Agriculture. It is a guide to food choices that we should be making every day in order to maintain a healthy diet.

The Food Guide Pyramid is a guideline as to what daily choices we should be making for ourselves to ensure that we receiving the nutrients and calories that we need to maintain a healthy weight.

A typical day would include 6-11 servings of bread, cereal, rice, and pasta.
Add to that 3-5 servings of Vegetables, 2-4 servings of fruit, 2-3 servings of meat, poultry, dry beans, eggs, or nuts and 2 to 3 servings of milk, yogurt or cheese. The only restrictions on this pyramid are to use fats, oils and sweet sparingly.

To see how well you are faring in feeding your body, write down everything you ate in one day, from waking up in the morning to going to bed at night. Yes, that includes how many teaspoons of sugar you put in your coffee and how many pads of butter you put on your biscuits.

Don't make any judgments (yet) on what you are writing down. Just jot down every morsel for one day. What you see staring back at you is a true mirror of what is going on in your body. Your daily diet will give you many clues as to your moods and experiences through the day.

Be sure to add the time you are eating every delectable morsel. You will soon learn a lot about yourself and may answer many of the questions you have as to why you are always tired.

If are not sure what constitutes a serving, then check the writing on the box, bag, or can. This information is always listed on the label on the product.

If you find yourself eating more than 1 serving, then be sure to count that as 2, or 3, servings. Actual serving sizes may surprise you as to how small they really are. When you start measuring out what constituents a serving size and see how many calories go with every serving size, you are on your way to making intelligent choices for your health.

The New Food Guide

Sample Menus for a 2000 Calorie Food Pattern

Averaged over a week, this seven day menu provides all of the recommended amounts of nutrients and food from each food group.
(Italicized foods are part of the dish or food that preceeds it.)

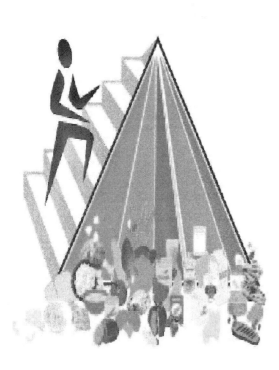

Food Group	Daily Average
GRAINS	Total Grains (oz eq) 6.0 Whole Grains 3.4 Refined Grains 2.6
VEGETABLES *	Total Veg* (cups) 2.6
FRUITS	Fruits (cups) 2.1
MILK	Milk (cups) 3.1
MEAT & BEANS	Meat/Beans (oz eq) 5.6
OILS	Oils (tsp/grams) 7.2 tsp/32.4 g

*Vegetable subgroups	(weekly totals)
Dk-Green Veg (cups)	3.3
Orange Veg (cups)	2.3
Beans/ Peas (cups)	3.0
Starchy Veg (cups)	3.4
Other Veg (cups)	6.6

Nutrient	Daily Average
Calories	1994
Protein, g	98
Protein, % kcal	20
Carbohydrate, g	264
Carbohydrate, % kcal	53
Total fat, g	67
Total fat, % kcal	30
Saturated fat, g	16
Saturated fat, % kcal	7.0
Monounsaturated fat, g	23
Polyunsaturated fat, g	23
Linoleic Acid, g	21
Alpha-linolenic Acid, g	1.1
Cholesterol, mg	207
Total dietary fiber, g	31
Potassium, mg	4715
Sodium, mg*	1948
Calcium, mg	1389
Magnesium, mg	432
Copper, mg	1.9
Iron, mg	21
Phosphorus, mg	1830
Zinc, mg	14
Thiamin, mg	1.9
Riboflavin, mg	2.5
Niacin Equivalents, mg	24
Vitamin B6, mg	2.9
Vitamin B12, mcg	18.4
Vitamin C, mg	190
Vitamin E, mg (AT)	18.9
Vitamin A, mcg (RAE)	1430
Dietary Folate Equivalents, mcg	558

* Starred items are foods that are labelled as no-salt-added, low-sodium, or low-salt versions of the foods. They can also be prepared from scratch with little or no added salt. All other foods are regular commercial products which contain variable levels of sodium. Average sodium level of the 7 day menu assumes no-salt-added in cooking or at the table.

MyPyramid Worksheet

MyPyramid.gov   Check how you did today and set a goal to aim for tomorrow

STEPS I\1A HEAlT HlER you

Write in Your Choices for Today	Food Group	Tip	Goal	List each food choice in its food group*	Estimate Your Total
_____ _____ _____	GRAINS	Make at least half your grains whole grains	6 ounce equivalents (1 ounce equivalent is about 1 slice bread, 1 cup dry cereal, or $1\frac{1}{2}$ cup rice or pasta)	_____ _____ _____	ounce equivalents
_____ _____	VEGETABLES	Try to have vegetables from several subgroups each day	$2\frac{1}{2}$ cups Subgroups: Dark Green, Orange, Starchy, Dry Beans and Peas, Other Veggies	_____ _____	cups
_____ _____	FRUITS	Make most choices cups fruit, not juice	2	_____ _____	cups
_____ _____	MILK	Choose fat-free or low fat most often	3 cups (1 $1\frac{1}{2}$ ounces cheese = 1 cup milkl	_____	cups
_____ _____ _____ _____	MEAT & BEANS	Choose lean meat and poultry. Vary your choices-more fish, beans, peas, nuts, and seeds	$5\frac{1}{2}$ ounce equivalents (1 ounce equivalent is 1 ounce meat, poultry or fish, 1 T. peanut butter, $1\frac{1}{2}$ ounce nuts, 1/4 cup dry beans or peas)	_____ — — — — — _____	ounce equivalents
_____ _____ _____	PHYSICAL ACTIVITY	Build more physical activity into your daily sugar- routine at home and work.	At least 30 minutes of moderate to vigorous activity a day, 10 minutes or more at a time.	'Some foods don't fit into any group. These "extras" may be mainly fat or limit your intake of these.	minutes

How did you do today?   0 Great   0 So-So   0 Not so Great

My food goal for tomorrow is: _____

My activity goal for tomorrow is: _____

MyPyramid Food Intake Pattern Calorie Levels

MyPyramid assigns Individuals to a calorie level based on their sex, age, and activity level.

The chart below identifies the calorie levels for males and females by age and activity level. Calorie levels are provided for each year of childhood, from 2-18 years, and for adults in 5-year increments.

	MALES				FEMALES		
Activity level	Sedentary*	Mod. active*	Active*	Activity level	Sedentary*	Mod. active*	Active*
AGE				AGE			
2	1000	1000	1000	2	1000	1000	1000
3	1000	1400	1400	3	1000	1200	1400
4	1200	1400	1600	4	1200	1400	1400
5	1200	1400	1600	5	1200	1400	1600
6	1400	1600	1800	6	1200	1400	1600
7	1400	1600	1800	7	1200	1600	1800
8	1400	1600	2000	8	1400	1600	1800
9	1600	1800	2000	9	1400	1600	1800
10	1600	1800	2200	10	1400	1800	2000
11	1800	2000	2200	11	1600	1800	2000
12	1800	2200	2400	12	1600	2000	2200
13	2000	2200	2600	13	1600	2000	2200
14	2000	2400	2800	14	1800	2000	2400
15	2200	2600	3000	15	1800	2000	2400
16	2400	2800	3200	16	1800	2000	2400
17	2400	2800	3200	17	1800	2000	2400
18	2400	2800	3200	18	1800	2000	2400
19-20	2600	2800	3000	19-20	2000	2200	2400
21-25	2400	2800	3000	21-25	2000	2200	2400
26-30	2400	2600	3000	26-30	1800	2000	2400
31-35	2400	2600	3000	31-35	1800	2000	2200
36-40	2400	2600	2800	36-40	1800	2000	2200
41-45	2200	2600	2800	41-45	1800	2000	2200
46-50	2200	2400	2800	46-50	1800	2000	2200
51-55	2200	2400	2800	51-55	1600	1800	2200
56-60	2200	2400	2600	56-60	1600	1800	2200
61-65	2000	2400	2600	61-65	1600	1800	2000
66-70	2000	2200	2600	66-70	1600	1800	2000
71-75	2000	2200	2600	71-75	1600	1800	2000
76 and up	2000	2200	2400	76 and up	1600	1800	2000

*Calorie levels are based on the Estimated Energy Requirements (EER) and activity levels from the Institute of Medicine Dietary Reference Intakes Macronutrients Report, 2002.
SEDENTARY = less than 30 minutes a day of moderate physical activity in addition to daily activities.
MOD. ACTIVE = at least 30 minutes up to 60 minutes a day of moderate physical activity in addition to daily activities.
ACTIVE = 60 or more minutes a day of moderate physical activity in addition to daily activities.

United StatesDepartment of Agriculture
Center for Nutrition Policy and Promotion
April 2005
CNPP-XX

For a free color, downloadable chart of your own, as shown on the previous pages, please go to: www.MyPyramid.gov .

The site also contains free downloadable information on starting a healthy diet, what constitutes a serving, and sample menu charts.

Also contained in the site is resource material for those in the health care industry for you to share with your clients. The recommendations listed are based on the Dietary Guidelines for Americans in 2005. The guidelines are recommended for the general public over the age of 2.

About the Author

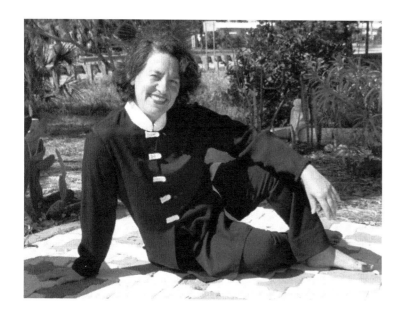

Francine Milford is a state and nationally certified massage therapist, personal trainer and energy worker. Francine has had a very long career in the Fitness Industry. Working for more than twenty years in a variety of sports and exercise related classes, she is also an avid walker and enjoys reading books on audio tape while bicycling or walking around the neighborhood.

She has achieved Aerobic certifications through the YMCA S.A.F.E. Aerobic Program, Water certifications through AEA Aquatics Exercise Association, Bench Stepping and Personal Training certifications through ESA Exercise Safety Association, and Personal Training through AFAA Aerobics Fitness Association of America, and Silver Sneakers certification (for work with seniors).

Francine has also received the Tai Chi for Arthritis certification having studied under Dr. Paul Lam, as well as, 180 hours of professional training in Tae Kwon Do. She has taught such classes as Kick Boxing, Bench Stepping, Low Impact Aerobics, High Impact Aerobics, Basic Floor and Senior Aerobics along with a variety of Water Aerobic, Weight Training and Ab Express classes.

As a personal trainer and fitness specialist, Francine has been hired to lead classes and workshops at offices, condo organizations, clubs and private groups. She is a continuing education provider for licensed massage therapist and athletic trainers. Having spent the last ten years working with the senior population, Francine has developed exercises that are both safe and effective for those with physical limitations.

If you liked this book, you may want to purchase one of Francine's other books such as Do~In, Qigong, H2O workouts, or Hand Therapy for Computer Users. For a list of other books, classes and workshops from Francine Milford, please check her websites at www.ReikiCenterofVenice.com or at www.FrancineMilford.com.

"Move with Mindfulness"

Francine

References

American College of Sport Medicine, Guidelines for Graded Exercise Testing and Exercise Prescription. Philadelphia: Lea and Febiger, 1995.

Hoeger, W.W.K. Principles and Labs for Physical Fitness and Wellness. Englewood, CO: Morton Publishing, 1999.

Phil, Mark Evans B., FNIMH, The Guide to Natural Therapies, Choosing and using natural methods for physical and mental well-being. Anness Publishing Limited 1996.

Wilson, Stanley D. Ph.D., QiGong for Beginners, Eight easy movements for vibrant Health, Rudra Press, 1997.

Websites

www.MyPyramid.gov

www.ReikiCenterofVenice.com

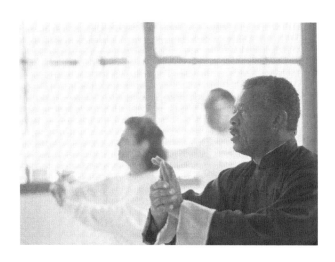

My Daily Journal

Use this journal to keep track of your progress doing the exercises in this manual. Begin at week one, day one and write down how you felt doing the exercises in this manual for the first time. Note your favorite movements and least favorite ones. How does your body feel right now, before you begin your exercise routine? How does it feel after the first week, the second week, etc.? Note any improvements you are sensing.

Week One

Day One

Day Two

Day Three

Day Four

Day Five

Day Six

Day Seven

Week Two

Day One

Day Two

Day Three

Day Four

Day Five

Day Six

Day Seven

Week Three

Day One

Day Two

Day Three

Day Four

Day Five

Day Six

Day Seven

Week Four

Day One

Day Two

Day Three

Day Four

Day Five

Day Six

Day Seven

Made in the USA
Middletown, DE
17 January 2023

22301655R00049